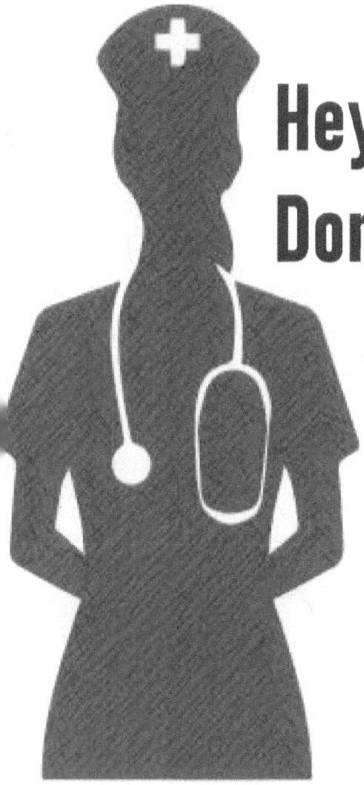

Hey, Nurse! Don't Mess This Up!

A Nurse Leader's Field Guide to People, Process, and Pressure

Tammy Dahl, DNP

"Every system is perfectly designed to get the results it gets."

Deming

Dedication

For Eric,

Thank you for your love, your patience, and your constant support.

And for every nurse

who has ever been called on, counted on, interrupted, stretched, and trusted to hold it all together.

Acknowledgments

This book exists because of a long career in nursing, leadership, and learning alongside others.

To my husband, Eric, thank you for your steady support, your patience, and your belief in me. You have been a constant source of strength, and I am deeply grateful.

To the many nurses, leaders, physicians, colleagues, and teams I have worked with over the years, thank you. You have taught me more than any formal education ever could.

You have shown me what leadership looks like under pressure, what teamwork looks like in imperfect circumstances, and what it means to keep going when the work is hard. Your examples, your challenges, and your commitment shaped the thinking behind this book.

To emerging nurse leaders, I wrote this with you in mind. Nursing leadership is demanding work. It asks for judgment, resilience, courage, and a willingness to keep learning. I hope that this book helps you feel less alone, more prepared, and more confident as you step into the responsibility of leading others.

Table of Contents

Quick Start (7 Days)

If you're a new leader—or you're leading through a rough season—don't try to "read the whole book." Use it like a field guide.

Day 1: Reset Your Leadership Nervous System

Read Chapter 1 and use one leadership phrase the same day. Pick one meeting and practice "Regulate → Clarify → Distribute ownership."

Day 2: Coach Defensiveness Without Escalation

Read Chapter 2. Choose one person/situation and use one line that lowers the temperature while holding the standard.

Day 3: Stop Triangulation

Read Chapter 4. Use one boundary leadership phrase to redirect the conversation back to the right person, the right forum, and the right next step.

Day 4: Run a Huddle That Produces Action

Read Chapter 6. In your next huddle, leave with at most 3 actions: the owner, the due date, and a follow-up point.

Day 5: Fix One Repeat Problem With a Rapid Cycle

Read Chapter 9. Choose one recurring issue and run a 30-minute rapid-cycle test with a 24-72-hour check-back.

Day 6: Fix One Handoff Seam

Read Chapter 11. Write a 'definition of done' for one handoff and pilot it for two weeks.

Day 7: Communicate With Structure

Read Chapter 14. Use the 4-part message: Why -> What is changing -> What stays the same -> What to do now. Repeat it consistently.

If you want the simplest rule for the week: choose one move, use it daily, and close the loop out loud.

Pocket Toolkit

These are the lines and micro-tools you can keep in your notes app. Use them exactly as written until they feel like yours.

10 Leadership Phrases That Stabilize the Moment

1. "I want to answer this well. Give me 10 minutes to confirm what we know and what we don't."
2. "Let's get specific: what's the top issue we need to solve in the next hour?"
3. "This number is a signal, not a grade. We're using it to learn and adjust—not to blame."
4. "Is this a decision, a recommendation, or information?"
5. "Who owns the next step, and what's the due date?"
6. "We're missing_____Here's the contingency for today, and here's how we prevent it tomorrow."
7. "Fix the pathway."
8. "Here's what we know today, what we don't know yet, and when you'll get the next update."
9. "I'll help us get to a solution, but I'm not going to own all of it. Who can take point?"
10. "When we're busy, we default to old habits. What would make the new way easier in the real workflow?"

Micro-Tools (Use in Under 2 Minutes)

Regulate: Exhale longer than you inhale x 5. Drop shoulders. Unclench jaw.

Clarify: Facts→ Impact → Next step. (No stories until you have facts.)

Close the loop: Decision + owner + due date + follow-up point (said out loud).

How to Keep This Alive Without Busy Work

Use one tool for 2 weeks. If it doesn't change behavior, retire it.

Who This Book is For (and Not For)

This book is for nurses who stepped into leadership and discovered that the hardest part isn't the clinical work—it's the human work: priorities, conflict, staffing realities, and decisions that don't come with a clean right answer.

This book is for you if you:

Went from being "the one who gets it done" to being responsible for the whole department or system getting it done.

Feel stress in your body before you even reach the unit/clinic (and then act like you're fine).

Care deeply about your people, yet still need to hold to a standard.

Want practical moves and leadership phrases—not theory.

Are tired of leading by adrenaline and want a steadier way.

This Book is Not For You If You:

Want a leadership memoir or a deep dive into academic models and theory.

Prefer vague inspiration over specific behaviors.

Believe leadership is about being liked more than being clear.

If you're busy, under-resourced, and trying not to mess it up, you're in the right place.

The Reader Promise

Use this book the way real leaders work: one chapter at a time, in the middle of real problems. If you do, you will get better at three things that matter most in healthcare leadership:

Regulating: staying steady enough to think when the room is stressed, and steady enough to help others think too.

Clarifying: turning chaos into a clear next step (facts -> impact -> decision). Simplify the complex. Make the work easier to see.

Closing loops: creating visible follow-through so your team experiences consistency instead of randomness.

You'll also leave with practical language for hard moments, lightweight tools to reduce rework, and ways to run huddles and meetings that actually move work forward.

Find the Chapter You Need (Index by Problem)

Use this when your day is on fire, and you don't have time to browse.

A staff member is defensive, reactive, or shuts down when coached. → Chapter 2

The team is stuck in blame, and nothing changes. → Chapter 3

People keep coming to me instead of talking to each other (triangulation). → Chapter 4

One informal "power center" is driving culture—for better or worse. → Chapter 5

Huddles drag on, turn into complaints, or don't produce action. → Chapter 6

Leaders are inconsistent; staff says, "It depends who's in charge." → Chapter 7

We have too many metrics and not enough improvement. → Chapter 8

The same problems repeat week after week. → Chapter 9

We roll out change, and it disappears under pressure. → Chapter 10

Cross-department friction is rising; work breaks at the seams. → Chapter 11

Handoffs are messy, and patient flow suffers. → Chapter 11

We're busy, but throughput is still broken (bottlenecks and queueing). → Chapter 12

Committees meet often, but decisions drift, and nothing gets executed. → Chapter 13

Rumors spread; messages get inconsistent; staff feel surprised. → Chapter 14

Don't Mess This Up

A practical leadership field guide for nurses who become leaders and suddenly inherit people problems, system problems, and a calendar with no mercy.

Introduction

If you are a nurse who stepped into leadership and immediately thought, This is a completely different job, you are not imagining it.

At the bedside, the work is demanding but visible. You assess, intervene, reassess, and move. In leadership, the work becomes less visible and far more diffuse. You inherit staffing strain, emotional spillover, unclear expectations, process failures, competing priorities, and the quiet pressure to look composed while all of it is happening at once.

The hardest part of the transition is not intelligence. It is identity. Many strong nurses become new leaders by being capable, dependable, and willing to carry more than their share. Those traits matter. But in leadership, over-carrying becomes a liability. The job is no longer to personally solve everything that lands in front of you. The job is to create enough clarity, steadiness, and follow-through that the team can function well under pressure.

That is why this book exists.

This is not a memoir, nor is it a theory-heavy leadership text. It is a field guide for real healthcare environments: short chapters, practical moves, language you can use out loud, and leadership habits that help you replace adrenaline with steadiness.

The core argument is simple: strong leadership is less about charisma and more about repeatable behaviors. Systems beat heroics. Clarity beats intensity. Follow-through beats good intentions.

Inside each chapter, you will see the same rhythm on purpose:

- what the problem looks like in real life
- why it matters
- what to do instead
- exact leadership language you can use
- a short checklist to help the change stick

Use the book for the full progression. Use it like a field manual if your day is already on fire. Either way, do not aim to master everything at once. Pick one move. Use it in the real workflow. Notice what changes.

You do not need a different personality to lead well. You need a steadier set of moves.

And yes, there is some humor in these pages. Healthcare is heavy work, and healthcare leadership is heavier. A little levity can help people breathe. But the humor here is never aimed at patients, families, or the dignity of the work. It is aimed at the predictable absurdities of systems under stress and at the very human things leaders do when they are trying too hard to hold everything together.

If you have ever walked to your car after a hard day and thought, I hope I handled that well, this book is for you.

The goal is not perfection. The goal is fewer preventable mistakes, faster recovery when they happen, and a team that experiences you as clear, steady, and useful when the pressure is on.

Let's get to work.

Part I

Stabilizing Yourself as a Leader

Chapter 1

Trying to Be the Calm And the Answer

The move from bedside nurse to leader rarely feels like a clean promotion. It feels more like being dropped into a role where the task list is made of people, tension, and unfinished problems.

One day, you know exactly what good work looks like. The next day, you are expected to make sense of staffing, conflict, throughput, physician concerns, patient complaints, and tomorrow's risk – often before you have had coffee.

That disorientation is normal. It does not mean you are failing. It means the work changed.

Leadership Moment

My First Real Leadership Wake-Up Call

What surprised me most about leadership was not the responsibility. It was the shift in what counted as competence.

At the bedside, I could see the work. In leadership, the work became interpretation, prioritization, containment, and follow-through.

I remember walking into an early leadership meeting and realizing no one was asking me to start an IV, assess a patient, or handle a medication issue. They were looking to me to make sense of staffing pressure, physician concerns, patient complaints, and the operational mess that was already unfolding.

I knew how to solve clinical problems. What I had not yet learned was how to hold people, business, and system problems without personally absorbing all of them.

That was the moment I began to understand the real job.

Leadership is not proving that you can carry everything.

Leadership is creating enough clarity and steadiness that the right work gets done by the right people at the right level.

The Friction (What This Looks Like in Real Life)

You walk into a unit, clinic, or huddle and immediately feel the emotional temperature.

Someone asks a question, and you feel pressure to answer instantly, because leaders are supposed to know.

You replay conversations in the shower and draft responses in your head at 2:00 a.m.

You over-function: fix, rescue, smooth, cover, and carry then wonder why you are exhausted and still behind.

You become the central nervous system for everybody else's anxiety.

Levity check: Leadership is one of the few jobs where 'How are you?' can be both a greeting and a threat assessment.

Why This Matters?

An anxious leader does not just feel bad; they feel anxious. An anxious leader changes the operating environment.

Teams start scanning you instead of the situation.

Decisions get rushed, blurred, or avoided.

You accidentally teach the team that the leader will absorb every loose end.

Your strongest people often carry extra until they burn out.

And you lose the very thing the role most needs from you: clarity.

The goal is not zero stress. The goal is to stop letting stress run the show.

The Move

Replace the reflex to instantly absorb and solve with a three-part sequence:

1) *Regulate first.*
2) *Clarify the second.*
3) *Distribute ownership.*

You do not need to fake certainty. You need enough steadiness to think before you react.

Step-by-Step (The 10-Minute Transition from Bedside Brain to Leader Brain)

Step 1: Do a 20-second reset before you walk in.

Put both feet on the floor. Drop your shoulders. Exhale longer than you inhale three times. Your body needs a signal: "We are safe enough to think."

Step 2: Name the weather—without dramatizing it.

Say what you're seeing in neutral language. This reduces gossip, mind-reading, and escalation.

Step 3: Separate "urgent" from "important."

Urgent gets a timebox. Important: get a plan. If everything is urgent, you're managing anxiety—not work.

Step 4: Decide what question this is.

Is this a decision, a data question, a workflow problem, or an emotion problem? Don't use one tool for all four.

Step 5: Create the next right step—small and owned.

Assign one owner, one deadline, one follow-up point. No owner = no action. No deadline = someday.

Step 6: Close the loop out loud.

Summarize what you decided, who owns what, and when you'll check back. This is how you build reliability.

Words You Can Use Monday (Leadership phrases)

Use these as written until they feel like yours. Clear beats clever.

When You Feel Pressure to Answer Immediately:

"I want to answer this well. Give me 10 minutes to confirm what we know and what we don't."

When The Room is Tense:

"I'm noticing we're carrying a lot today. Let's get specific: what's the main issue we need to solve in the next hour?"

When Someone Wants You to Fix it:

"I'll help us get to a solution, but I'm not going to own all of it. Who's closest to the work and can take point?"

When People are Spiraling into Stories:

"Let's pause. What are the facts? What's the impact? What do we need next?"

When You Don't Know (And Your Ego is Sweating):

"I don't know yet—and I'm going to find out. Here's what I can commit to by the end of the day."

When You Need To Slow The Pace:

"We're moving fast, and speed can create mistakes. Let's timebox this and make a clean decision."

When You Need Boundaries Without Guilt:

"I can do A or B today. I can't do both well. Which is the priority?"

Pocket Checklist

- ☐ Reset your body before you walk in (exhale longer than inhale).
- ☐ Name the weather neutrally (no drama, no denial).
- ☐ Ask: Is this urgent, important, or both?
- ☐ Define the problem in one sentence.
- ☐ Choose the tool: decision/data/workflow/emotion.
- ☐ Assign one owner (not "we").
- ☐ Set one deadline (not "soon").
- ☐ Document one sentence: decision + owner + due date + follow-up point.
- ☐ Close the loop out loud.
- ☐ Follow through on what you said you would (this is how trust is built).
- ☐ In your daily huddle or end-of-day wrap, ask: "What did we assign ownership to today—and did we close the loop?"

Mini Tool: The 2-Minute Nervous System Reset (Use Before Hard Conversations)

This is not "self-care." This is operational readiness.

1. **Exhale for 6 seconds.** Inhale for 4 seconds. Repeat 5 times.

2. **Unclench your jaw.** Drop your tongue from the roof of your mouth.
3. **Name three facts in the room (grounding):** "I'm in my office. It's Tuesday. I have time to think."
4. **Choose your intention:** "I will be clear and kind."
5. Walk in with your first sentence ready (use a leadership phrase above).

If You Only Remember One Thing

Your job is not to carry everyone's stress. Your job is to create clarity and follow through under stress.

You'll still feel anxiety sometimes. The difference is: you won't let it run the conversation.

Chapter 2

Coaching Defensiveness Without Triggering a War

Defensiveness is rarely about you. It's usually fear wearing armor. The mess-up is meeting armor with force—or tiptoeing around it until it runs the unit.

Leadership Moment

Graduate school taught me the language of leadership. The emergency department taught me how hard it is to use that language in a real conversation.

My MSN program covered core leadership competencies: strategic planning, communication and collaboration, healthcare finance, quality improvement, and navigating complex healthcare systems.

Those frameworks were valuable. They gave me a mental model for how organizations function.

But the real test of leadership didn't show up in a classroom.

It showed up in a coaching conversation.

When I was serving as the director of an emergency department in California, I worked with a strong nursing manager and experienced charge nurses. One day, I needed to address a situation where expectations hadn't been met.

As soon as the issue came up, the response came quickly—explanations, barriers, and reasons why the situation wasn't really their responsibility.

For a moment, the conversation began drifting toward debate. I could feel the tension rising, that familiar moment where coaching can easily turn into an argument.

In that moment, I realized something important: leadership frameworks are helpful, but they only matter if you can use them when the room gets uncomfortable.

So, I paused and asked a simple question:

"Before we talk about the barriers, what part of this do you own?"

The room got quiet.

That question changed the direction of the conversation. Instead of defending the past, we began talking about the next step.

That was One of My Early Leadership Lessons:

Coaching isn't about winning the argument. It's about helping someone stay open long enough to take ownership.

The Friction (What's Happening in Real Life)

You give feedback. The recipient reacts quickly—explains, justifies, blames, or points at everyone else's role. The conversation shifts from focusing on improvement to a debate. Over time, staff learn not to raise concerns, peers stop working together, and results stall because accountability is always "shared" but never truly owned.

Why This Matters

Defensiveness isn't an interpersonal issue—it's an execution problem.

It blocks learning ("I'm fine, the other unit is the problem").

It erodes trust ("feedback isn't safe here").

It kills speed (everything becomes an argument instead of a plan).

It trains the team to walk on eggshells or route around the leader.

Your goal isn't to "make them feel good." Your goal is to build a leader who can stay open under pressure and own the outcomes.

The Move (What To Do)

Step 1: Set the stage (30 seconds)

Start with purpose + boundaries so the conversation doesn't drift into defense.

Say:

"I intend to help you be successful and strengthen outcomes in your area."

"I'm going to be specific. We'll focus on what's in your control and what you'll do next."

"This isn't about fault. It's about ownership and follow-through."

Step 2: Lead with observable facts + impact (60 seconds)

Avoid labels ("defensive," "immature," "not accountable"). Use behavior + impact.

Template:

When (what occurred): ______________________________ ,

I observed: _______________________________________ ,

resulting in (Impact):______________________________ ,

Expectation:______________________________ .

Example:

"When the missed deadline came up in the huddle, you listed barriers and named two departments, but you didn't state your recovery plan. The team was left unclear on the next steps. From now on, I need you to close with what you own and the recovery plan by the end of the day."

Step 3: Interrupt the defensive spiral early (the "pause and pivot")

When they begin explaining/blaming, don't argue. Redirect.

Say:

"I'm going to stop you—not because those factors aren't real, but because this is skipping ownership."

"We can discuss contributors later. Right now: what do you own, and what will you do next?"

Step 4: Separate context from accountability (repeatable rule)

Rule: "Context is welcome. Accountability is required."

Say:

"That's helpful context—and you still own the outcome."

"Given those constraints, what's your plan?"

Step 5: Install a new default response (practice it)

Defensive leaders or employees often don't have an alternative leadership phrase. Give them one.

The new first response (non-negotiable):

"I hear you."

"Let me reflect."

"Here's what I'll do."

Then they can add context after ownership.

Step 6: Close with commitments (or it didn't happen)

Defensiveness fades when accountability becomes routine.

Close With:

"What are your 3 actions, by when?"

"How will you update me?"

"What help do you need—and what are you doing regardless?"

Document it in a short recap.

The leadership phrases (use these word-for-word)

When you sense defensiveness starting

"I'm going to pause you. I'm hearing an explanation before ownership."

"I'm not questioning your intent. I'm addressing impact."

"Let's park the 'why' and go to 'what next.'"

"We can validate the barriers and still require a plan."

When they blame others

"Those factors may be true. What part is yours to own?"

"If you couldn't change anyone else, what would you do?" [My Favorite!!]

"What conversation do you need to lead, and by when?"

"I'm open to cross-functional issues—after we hear your recovery plan."

When they argue, the feedback

"You don't have to agree with me to act on the gap."

"Let's not debate the past. Let's decide the next standard."

"What's one piece of this you can accept as useful?"

"Help me understand—then tell me what you're going to do."

When they shut down (silence, tears, stonewalling)

"I can see this is landing hard. I'm not attacking you."

"Would you like 10 minutes to regroup, then come back with a plan?"

"I'm going to stay with this because you're capable—and this matters."

When you need to name the pattern directly

"Can I share an observation about how feedback is landing?"

"When feedback is less than positive, you move quickly to defending. The risk is that we miss learning, and others experience low accountability. Are you open to practicing a different response?"

The standard you're installing

"Your first response needs to be: 'I hear you. Here's what I own. Here's what I'll do next.' Context comes second."

Pocket Checklist (Keep It To 10)

Before the conversation:

- ☐ Choose one specific example (time/place/behavior)
- ☐ Know the impact (outcome/culture/safety/speed)
- ☐ Decide the expectation (what "good" looks like)

During:

- ☐ Open with intent + container
- ☐ State facts + impact (no labels)
- ☐ Interrupt defensiveness early ("pause and pivot")
- ☐ Ask for ownership: "What do you own?"
- ☐ Require a plan: "What will you do by when?"

Close:

- ☐ Confirm 2–3 commitments with dates
- ☐ Set follow-up cadence (check-in date/time)

Red Flags (what not to do)

Don't over-explain or "sell" the feedback (it invites debate).

Don't accept "we" ownership when the role requires "I" ownership.

Don't end with "Let's keep an eye on it" (that's code for no accountability).

Don't let them recruit you into blaming others.

If You Only Remember One Thing

Defensiveness is a stress response, not a cue for you to get louder. Slow the moment down, separate context from accountability, and leave with a clear next step the other person owns.

Chapter 3

Turning Blame into Ownership (Without a Fight)

When things go sideways, the human brain wants a culprit. Leadership is helping the team trade "Who did this?" for "What do we do next?"—without sounding like a poster.

The Friction (What's Happening in Real Life)

When something goes wrong—missed deadlines, patient complaints, workflow breakdowns—some leaders reflexively explain, point outward, or dilute accountability by making it "we" and "they." It's rarely malicious; it's usually self-protection. But the impact is predictable: problems repeat, trust erodes, and the team learns that accountability is optional.

Why This Matters

Blame feels like motion, but it's avoidance.

It slows improvement because energy goes into defending instead of fixing

- It damages teamwork ("I'll protect myself first")
- It teaches staff to hide errors and soften the truth
- It creates chronic excuses and low reliability

Ownership is the opposite of blame. Ownership says: "I will lead the fix."

The Move (What To Do)

Step 1: Separate "contributors" from "owner of the fix"

Many issues have multiple contributors. But every issue needs one owner for the recovery plan.

Say it plainly:

"Many things may have contributed. One person still owns the recovery plan."

Step 2: Use the "Context is welcome; accountability is required" rule

You don't deny reality—you refuse to let reality become an excuse.

Say:

"Those barriers are real—and you still own the outcome."

"Given that context, what's your plan?"

Step 3: Make ownership visible with three required sentences

Teach a simple structure. Require it every time.

The Ownership Triple (non-negotiable):

- "Here's what happened (facts)."
- "Here's what I own."
- "Here's what I will do by when."

If they can't say #2 and #3, they're not owning it.

Step 4: Redirect blame in real time (without arguing)

Don't debate their narrative. pivot.

The redirect sequence:

Validate briefly: "I hear that."

Reset focus: "Now—what do you own?"

Require plan: "What's next, by when?"

Step 5: Hold the line on roles and expectations

If their role owns the outcome, don't accept "shared responsibility" as a hiding place.

Say:

"I agree others have roles. In this seat, you own the outcome."

"If you need support, ask for it—don't outsource accountability."

Step 6: Close with commitments + follow-up

Ownership only becomes culture when it's routine and visible.

Close with:

"Summarize your plan: actions, owners, due times."

"When will you update me?"

"What's the escalation path if blocked?"

The Leadership Phrases (Use These Word-For-Word)

To stop blaming quickly

"I hear the barriers. Now tell me what you own."

"We can map contributors later. First: Who owns the recovery plan?"

"Let's separate explanation from action. What's the next step?"

"If you couldn't change anyone else, what would you do?"

To reframe accountability without shaming

"This isn't about fault. It's about ownership and follow-through."

"Context is helpful—and we still need a plan."

"You don't have to carry it alone, but you do have to carry it forward."

To require specificity

"What does 'fix it' mean specifically—what will be different?"

"By when, and how will we measure it?"

"Who needs to be informed today?"

To handle repeated excuses

"I'm noticing a pattern of explanation without commitment."

"What commitment are you willing to make right now?"

"This has come up before—what will be different this time?"

To move from 'we' to 'I.'

"I'm going to ask you to use 'I' language: what will you do?"

"Where will you personally intervene this week?"

Pocket Checklist

- ☐ Start with facts (no stories)
- ☐ Identify impact (safety / flow / workforce / experience / finance)
- ☐ Ask: "Who owns the recovery plan?"
- ☐ Require the Ownership Triple (facts / I own / I will)
- ☐ Convert barriers into a plan (next step + due time)
- ☐ Define escalation if blocked
- ☐ Close with 2–3 dated commitments
- ☐ Document commitments (short recap)
- ☐ Follow up within 7 days
- ☐ Close the loop with stakeholders

Red Flags (What Not To Do)

Don't let the conversation become a trial ("who's at fault?").

Don't accept vague commitments ("we'll work on it").

Don't allow "shared responsibility" to replace clear ownership.

Don't let the loudest voice define reality—anchor in facts.

If You Only Remember One Thing

Do not spend your leadership energy deciding who to blame first. Name the facts, assign the fix owner, and require a dated plan.

Chapter 4

Getting Stuck in the Middle (Triangulation & Conflict Containment)

If you feel like the emotional sponge of your department, congratulations—you've been triangulated. The fix isn't working harder. The fix is changing the flow of conversations.

Conflict Containment and Triangulation

One day, the ER charge nurse approached me, clearly frustrated. She had just spoken with the Imaging Lead, who had asked the ER to transport patients to and from imaging during that shift.

The charge nurse said, "They don't understand what it's like for us. We don't have time to transport patients. That's their job, not ours. I'm done talking with him—they always try to avoid work. Will you talk to him and tell him this isn't going to work?"

In other words, she was asking me to step in and carry the message.

I paused and asked a simple question:

"Did you ask the Imaging Lead why they couldn't follow the process today?"

She said no. She was so frustrated that as soon as he made the request, she turned and walked away.

So I asked a second question:

"There might be something different about today that led him to make that request. What could you do next?"

Then I added something important.

You're both leaders of your respective areas. If I intervene and pass messages between you, it won't resolve the issue—it will only escalate the conflict.

The charge nurse paused briefly before saying, "You're right. I'll go back and talk with him."

Later, she came back and told me the rest of the story. Imaging had unexpectedly lost a staff member mid-shift, and they were trying to keep patient care moving.

That moment reinforced a leadership lesson for me: When leaders carry messages between frustrated people, conflict grows. When leaders encourage direct conversation, solutions appear.

The Friction (What's Happening in Real Life)

A conflict starts between two people or two departments. Instead of addressing it directly, one (or both) begin recruiting allies:

"Can you talk to them?"

"So, you know..."

"Everyone is saying..."

"I don't want to make a big deal, but..."

Soon you're in the middle—carrying messages, soothing emotions, and trying to keep the peace. Meanwhile, the original conflict grows teeth, spreads, and becomes a cultural issue. This is triangulation: conflict moves sideways rather than being resolved.

Why This Matters

Triangulation feels like help, but it creates:

rumors and distorted facts

sides and loyalty tests

avoidance (people stop speaking directly)

leader overload (you become the messenger and therapist)

slow execution (work stalls while people argue)

Your goal is not to eliminate conflict. Your goal is to keep conflict where it belongs and move it toward resolution.

The Move (What To Do)

Step 1: Name the rule of engagement

Make this a standard in your leadership culture:

Rule: "We speak to the person, not about the person." Exception: Safety, harassment, discrimination, retaliation, or policy violations (those come to you/HR immediately).

Step 2: Stop accepting "drive-by complaints"

A drive-by complaint is information given without a request, ownership, or intention to resolve it directly.

Your response:

"What do you want to have happen?"

"Have you told them directly?"

"What's your next step?"

If they won't act, don't adopt it.

Step 3: Use the "two options" to redirect (fast and calm)

When someone brings you a conflict that belongs between peers:

Option A: "I'll support you in addressing this directly."

Option B: "If you want me involved, we'll do a joint conversation—no side conversations."

This removes the intermediary role.

Step 4: Require a direct conversation plan

If they claim they "can't" talk to the person, you coach it.

Plan elements:

What they will say (facts + impact + request)

When will they say it (date/time)

What "resolved" looks like

Step 5: Facilitate only when necessary—and facilitate correctly

If it's stuck, high-emotion, or cross-departmental, you step in as a facilitator.

Your facilitation structure (20–30 minutes):

Purpose: "We're here to resolve, not relive."

Facts: each person states facts only

Impact: each states the impact

Needs: each state what they need going forward, what they are looking for

Agreement: decide next steps, owners, and due times

Close: how you'll follow up

Step 6: Contain repeated conflict with clear boundaries

When a pattern repeats, it needs a standard.

Examples:

- *handoff agreements*
- *role clarity*
- *escalation paths*
- *meeting norms*
- *decision rights*

The leadership phrases (use these word-for-word)

When someone tries to triangulate you

"Have you talked to them directly?"

"What's your ask—what do you want to happen?"

"I'm not going to carry messages. I will support a direct conversation."

"If you want me involved, we'll meet together—no side channels."

When they say they're afraid to address it

"What's the risk you're worried about?"

"Let's plan your first two sentences and the specific request."

"I'll help you prepare, but you need to lead the conversation."

When someone wants you to "fix " another person

"I can't fix what I haven't heard directly from both sides."

"I'm happy to facilitate—after you've attempted a direct conversation."

"What have you already tried?"

During a facilitated conversation (keep it contained)

- "Facts only—no labels, no mind-reading."
- "Say what you need going forward in one sentence."
- "What are we agreeing to today—owner and due time?"
- "We're not deciding who's right; we're deciding what we'll do."

When the conflict goes public (gossip)

"If you have a concern, bring it to the person or to me—not to the hallway."

"We don't do rumor leadership here."

Pocket Checklist

- ☐ Identify if it's a true escalation (safety/policy) vs peer conflict
- ☐ Ask: "Have you addressed it directly?"
- ☐ Require an ask: "What do you want to happen?"
- ☐ Use the two-option redirect (direct talk or joint meeting)
- ☐ Coach the direct conversation (facts, impact, request)
- ☐ Set a date/time for the conversation
- ☐ Facilitate only if stuck/high-impact
- ☐ Use the 6-step facilitation structure
- ☐ Document agreements (who/what/by when)
- ☐ Follow up in 7 days and close the loop

Red Flags (What Not To Do)

- Don't become the messenger—you'll create dependency and resentment.
- Don't take action based on one-sided stories.
- Don't allow "everyone is saying" to substitute for facts.
- Don't force "be nice"— force clarity, respect, and agreements.

Part II

Running the Daily Work

Chapter 5

Letting Informal Power Run the Show

Every team has power centers. Some build culture. Some blow it up. Your job isn't to "win" against influence—it's to make it visible, useful, and accountable.

Power Centers and Disruptive Influence (Without Losing the Relationship)

The Friction (What's Happening in Real Life)

Every organization has "power centers"—people with outsized influence due to tenure, reputation, referral volume, technical expertise, political capital, or sheer confidence. Sometimes they are constructive.

Sometimes they are disruptive, using intimidation, side deals, undermining leaders, public criticism, disrespect toward staff, refusal to follow agreed processes, or "special rules" that weaken fairness. I see this repeatedly in astute surgeons. My sister experienced this while working in law firms.

Leaders Often Freeze Because They Think:

- "We need them."
- "They'll retaliate."
- "They're too influential to confront."
- "If I push back, I'll lose the relationship."

Why This Matters

Unchecked disruptive influence quietly rewrites your culture:

- Staff stop speaking up
- standards become optional
- Other leaders copy the behavior
- Teamwork collapses into politics
- Patient care and flow become inconsistent

This is not a personality problem. It's a governance and standards problem.

The Move (What To Do)

Step 1: Anchor to a shared non-negotiable

You need one "north star" that no one can argue with.

Use one of these:

- Patient safety and reliable care (why we are in healthcare)
- Respectful behavior toward staff (organizational values)
- Agreed access/ flow standards (best practice)
- Compliance requirements (the must-haves)
- Fairness and transparency (code of conduct)

Say:

"We can debate preferences. We can't debate patient safety, respectful conduct, or agreed-upon standards." Agreed-upon standards are established by governing committees, such as the Medical Executive Committee or the Surgery Committee.

Step 2: Prepare before you confront (the 5-part prep)

Power centers win when you come unprepared.

Facts (specific examples, dates, witnesses if needed)

Impact (patient flow, staff retention, safety, culture)

Standard (what should happen instead)

Ask (specific behavior change)

Boundary (what happens if it continues)

Step 3: Have the conversation privately, quickly, and directly

Use the calmest tone you can. Don't overtalk.

Structure (7 minutes):

Intent: "I want you to be successful here, and I value your contribution."

- **Facts:** "Here's what I observed..."
- **Impact:** "Here's the impact..."
- **Standard:** "Here's what must happen going forward..."
- **Commitment:** "Can you agree to that?"
- **Boundary:** "If it happens again, here's the next step..."

Step 4: Convert influence into ownership (when appropriate)

When someone has strong opinions, they often want control. Give them a constructive lane—without giving them veto power.

Say:

"If you want a different outcome, I'm open to you helping design the solution. The standard still applies while we improve it."

Step 5: Stop special rules (this is where culture is won)

Power centers often succeed through exceptions.

Rule: exceptions must be visible, time-limited, justified, and approved through the same path for everyone.

No private deals.

Step 6: Use "two-level" accountability: behavior + system

You address conduct AND system conditions.

- **Behavior:** tone, respect, adherence to agreed process
- **System:** unclear handoffs, bad policies, inadequate capacity, poor scheduling design

This keeps it fair and credible.

Step 7: If it's persistent, escalate formally

Disruptive behavior that harms staff or safety is not a style; it's not a personality trait. It's a risk.

Escalation Options (Depending on Your Structure):

- Involve CMO/Chief of Staff
- Professional conduct policy pathway
- Peer review/medical staff bylaws (for physicians)
- HR performance management (for employed leaders)
- Documented expectations and follow-up dates
- The leadership phrases (use these word-for-word)

Opening a Hard Conversation With an Influential Person

"I value your contribution here, and I want us aligned."

"I'm going to be direct because this matters to patients and staff."

"Here's what I observed... and here's the impact."

Naming the Standard Without Arguing

"This is the standard going forward."

"You may disagree, but this is not optional."

"We can improve the process—after we follow the current agreement."

When Intimidation or Disrespect Occurs

"I'm going to stop you. That tone isn't acceptable here."

"We can be frustrated and still be respectful."

"If this continues, I will end the meeting and we'll reconvene with ____."

When They Push for an Exception

"I'm not doing side deals."

"If an exception is needed, we'll make it visible and time-limited."

"What's the clinical or operational reason, and what's the mitigation?"

Converting Criticism into Ownership

"If you see a better way, I want your help designing it."

"What are you willing to own by when?"

Closing with Boundaries

"Can you commit to this standard?"

"If this happens again, the next step is a"

Pocket Checklist

- ☐ Identify the non-negotiable anchor (safety/ respect/ standard)
- ☐ Gather 2–3 specific facts (date/ time/ behavior)
- ☐ Define the impact (culture, staff, flow, safety)
- ☐ Define the expected standard (behavior/ process)
- ☐ Decide your clear ask (what must change)
- ☐ Plan your boundary (what happens next if repeated)
- ☐ Meet privately; calm tone; short and direct
- ☐ Get a commitment (yes/ no)
- ☐ Document the standard and follow-up date
- ☐ Escalate if repeated—don't renegotiate boundaries

Red Flags (What Not To Do)

Don't confront without facts—power centers will spin and win.

Don't wait until you're angry—address early while calm.

Don't trade standards for peace—others will watch and conclude standards are optional.

Don't let "we need them" override patient safety, staff safety, and dignity. [This tends to occur with physicians whom the health system values].

Sidebar: The 4 Types of Power (and how to respond)

Expert Power (Skills/ Knowledge) → Respect expertise, require respectful behavior

Tenure Power (History/ Relationships) → Honor contribution, enforce standards equally

Volume Power (revenue/ referrals) → Align to system outcomes, stop special rules

Social Power (Alliances/ Influence) → Keep decisions transparent and documented

Mini Tool: Influential Stakeholder Alignment Plan

Name/Role: ______________________________

Influence Type: ☐ Expert ☐ Tenure ☐ Volume ☐ Social

- Non-negotiable Standard:

  ____

  ____

- Observed Behaviors (Facts):

  ____

  ____

- Impact:

  ____

  ____

- My Ask (Specific Change):

  ____

  ____

- What I Can Offer (Constructive Lane):

  ____

  ____

- Boundary If Repeated:

____

____

- Follow-up Date/ Time:

____

____

- Escalation Path (if needed):

____

____

Chapter 6

Turning Huddles into Story Time

A huddle is not group therapy or a status update. It's a brief, focused moment where you foster clarity, ownership, and progress—especially on tough days. It can start with a positive patient story or a special shout-out to an employee who went above and beyond.

The Friction (What's Happening in Real Life)

Translation: If it doesn't end with an owner and a due time, it's story time.

Many huddles drift into status updates, storytelling, or problem-listing with no owner. People leave with the same confusion they arrived with, and "we talked about it" becomes the substitute for execution. Over time, the huddle becomes optional, then pointless, then a culture signal: we meet, but we don't move.

Why This Matters

A good huddle is a daily reliability engine. It surfaces risks early (before they become events)

- Aligns priorities fast
- Creates clear ownership
- Reduces interruptions later
- Builds a cadence of accountability without drama

The huddle isn't a meeting. It's a daily operational reset.

The Move (What To Do)

The 10-minute structure (non-negotiable)

Standing. At the same time. Same place. Same scoreboard. Same closing.

Minute 0–1: *Start on time, state purpose*

"This is a 10-minute operational reset: safety, flow, staffing, today's barriers, and who owns what."

Minute 1–3: *Safety & quality (today's risks)*

Any overnight events/near misses? Any high-risk patients or processes today?

"What are we watching closely today?"

Minutes 3–5: *Staffing & capacity*

staffing gaps, skill mix, breaks coverage, surges expected

"Where are we thin and what's our mitigation?"

Minutes 5–7: *Flow & throughput; bottlenecks (admissions, discharges, diagnostics, transfers, procedure start times) "Where will the day get stuck?"*

Minutes 7–9: *Barriers needing escalation*

Only items that require help beyond the team's control

Each barrier must have: owner + next step + due time

Minutes 9–10: *Close with commitments*

"Here are the actions, owners, and times. Any critical handoffs before we break?"

The rule that keeps huddles from turning into therapy

No story without a decision.

If someone starts explaining, you redirect:

"What do you need, and what's the next step?"

"Who owns it, by when?"

Keep the "parking lot" small and real.

Anything requiring discussion goes to a separate problem-solving slot (A3, mini-rapid improvement, 15–30 minutes). The huddle identifies and assigns—it doesn't solve everything.

The leadership phrases (use these word-for-word)

To keep it tight

"Pause—what's the ask and who owns the next step?"

"What's the decision we need today?"

"If it can't be acted on today, it goes to the parking lot."

"Let's take that offline—what's the immediate mitigation right now?"

To prevent blame and keep ownership

"What do we control, and what's our plan?"

"Context noted. Now: owner, action, time."

"Who is the single accountable owner?"

To manage escalation cleanly

"Is this within our control? If not, what's the escalation path?"

"What do you need from me specifically?"

"By when will we know this is resolved?"

To close strong

"Say your commitment back: what will you do by what time?"

"If you're blocked, notify by ____ so we can pivot."

Pocket Checklist

Huddle Setup

- ☐ Same time/location; stand if possible
- ☐ Visible scoreboard (3–7 metrics max)
- ☐ Attendance: core roles only (others as needed)

During

- ☐ Start on time; restate purpose
- ☐ Safety risks first
- ☐ Staffing/capacity next
- ☐ Flow bottlenecks next
- ☐ Barriers: owner + next step + due time
- ☐ Park anything that needs discussion

Close

- ☐ Read back actions/owners/times
- ☐ Confirm critical handoffs

Red Flags (What Not To Do)

Don't let it become a status meeting ("everyone go around the room").

Don't allow problem dumping without ownership.

Don't exceed 10 minutes—long huddles train people to avoid them.

Don't track 20 metrics—use a small scoreboard tied to decisions.

Sidebar: The Huddle Scoreboard (simple and effective)

Keep it to 3–7 measures, visible, and tied to action. Examples:

Safety: falls, near-miss count, high-risk patients flagged

Flow: discharges by noon, pending diagnostics, OR start-time reliability

Workforce: call-outs, breaks, compliance risk, sitter needs

Experience: top service recovery issues today

Mini tool: Huddle Action Log (One Line Per Action)

Date: ________________________________

Barrier: ______________________________

Owner: ______________________________

Next step: ____________________________

Due time: ____________________________

Escalation needed? Y/N

Status: ☐ Open / ☐ Done / ☐ Rolled

Leader's Huddle Pledge

(A short commitment I can share with my team)

I will lead (or ensure) a daily huddle that strengthens reliability, protects safety, and creates clear ownership.

I commit that our huddles will be:

On Time and Time-boxed: 10 minutes, standing when possible.

Purpose-driven: a daily operational reset—not a status meeting.

Safe and Respectful: issues are raised without blame; we focus on solutions.

Action-oriented: no problem dumping—every barrier ends with an owner and due time.

Transparent: our scoreboard is visible and tied to decisions.

Accountable: we read back commitments and follow up on what we said we'd do.

Our Standard Huddle Close will be:

"Here are the actions, owners, and due times. If you're blocked, escalate by _____. Thank you."

Leader Name: ______________________________

Role/Department: ___________________________

Date: _____________________________________

One-page Printable: 10-Minute Huddle Agenda + Action Log (Word-ready)

DEPARTMENT/UNIT: _________________________

DATE: ___________________________________

HUDDLE TIME: _____________________________

LEAD: ___________________________________

10-Minute Huddle Agenda (check as completed)

☐ 0–1 min | Purpose: "10-minute operational reset: safety, staffing, flow, barriers, owners."

☐ 1–3 min | Safety/Quality risks today: (events/near misses, high-risk patients/processes)

☐ 3–5 min | Staffing/Capacity: (call-outs, skill mix, break coverage, surge risks)

- ☐ 5–7 min | Flow/Throughput: (bottlenecks, pending diagnostics, discharges, start-time risks)
- ☐ 7–9 min | Barriers + escalation: (only items needing help beyond team control)
- ☐ 9–10 min | Read-back: actions, owners, due times + critical handoffs

Today's Scoreboard (3–7 metrics max)

____

Today: _______

Target: _______

____

Today: _______

Target: _______

____

Today: _______

Target: _______

____

Today: _______

Target: _______

____

Today: _______

Target: _______

____

Today: _______

Target: _______

____

Today: _______

Target: _______

Huddle Action Log (one line per action)

Close (leadership phrase)

Actions/Owners/Due Times read back?

☐ Yes ☐ No

Critical handoffs confirmed?

☐ Yes ☐ No

If blocked, escalate to:

____

by ______________ (time)

Chapter 7

Calling it "Standard Work" and Watching Everyone Roll Their Eyes

Leader standard work isn't about turning humans into robots. It's about reducing decision fatigue, so your team gets consistency rather than personality-based leadership.

Leader Standard Work (Lightweight but Real)

The Friction (What's Happening in Real Life)

Translation: Standard work isn't about controlling adults. It's about making the best way the easiest way.

When leaders don't have a consistent operating rhythm, the day runs them. They spend time reacting—answering texts, putting out fires, jumping into staffing gaps—then wonder why the same problems keep returning. Staff experiences this as unpredictability: "It depends on who's on and how busy it is." Reliability suffers because leadership attention isn't reliable.

Why This Matters

Leader Standard Work (LSW) is how you make leadership dependable.

It prevents drift (standards and processes slowly decay)

It catches risk early (before events, complaints, overtime spikes)

It turns "busy" into disciplined execution

It creates fairness (everyone gets the same leadership support)

LSW is not bureaucracy. It's the smallest set of habits that protects outcomes.

The Move (What To Do)

Step 1: Standardize the "critical few" (not everything)

Pick 5–7 must-dos that directly protect safety, flow, workforce, and follow-through. If it doesn't protect an outcome, it's not standard work.

The critical few usually include:

daily huddle attendance/ leadership

visibility rounding (patients + staff)

review of key metrics/ risks

barrier removal + escalation follow-through

coaching/ feedback touchpoint

handoff and planning (today/ tomorrow)

Step 2: Build a simple cadence: Daily / Weekly / Monthly

Keep LSW short, visible, and repeatable.

Daily (20–40 Minutes Total, Split up):

- Huddle (10 min)
- Rounding (10–15 min)
- Action-log follow-up (5–10 min)
- 1 coaching touchpoint (2–5 min)

Weekly (30–60 minutes):

- Review the top 3–5 recurring barriers and pick one to fix
- Check staffing patterns, overtime, quality signals, complaints
- Confirm improvement work is moving (not "tracked")

Monthly (60–90 minutes):

- "Stop/ start/ continue" on operations
- Skills mix and retention themes
- Standard work audit: what's slipping and why

Step 3: Use a "standard question" leadership phrase during rounding

Rounding isn't friendliness. It's operational sensing.

Ask the same questions so patterns emerge:

- "What's getting in the way of great care today?"
- "Where are we at risk?"
- "What's one thing we should fix this week?"
- "Is there anything you've raised that hasn't been resolved?"

Step 4: Make follow-through visible (the credibility engine)

Nothing builds trust like closing loops.

Rule: Every barrier has:

- Owner
- Next Step
- Due Time
- Close-the-loop Message Back to the Person/ Team

Step 5: Keep it "lightweight but real"

LSW fails when it becomes a checklist no one uses. Use a one-page tracker that lives with you.

The leadership phrases (use these word-for-word)

To protect the cadence

- "If it's important, it gets a cadence. If it has no cadence, it's not important yet."
- "I'm going to be consistent, not perfect. Consistency wins."
- "I'm not available for new work until we close yesterday's commitments."

During Rounding (to Surface Real Issues)

- "What's the one thing that would make today safer or smoother?"
- "Where are we most likely to get stuck today?"
- "What have you raised before that still isn't fixed?"
- "What workaround are we relying on right now?"
- To prevent problem dumping
- "What do you need from me specifically?"
- "Who owns the next step, and when will it be done?"
- "If we can't solve it today, what's the mitigation today?"
- To close loops (build trust)
- "Here's what we did, what's next, and when you'll see it."
- "If this isn't better by Friday, we'll escalate to____."

Pocket Checklist

Daily

- ☐ Attend/lead the 10-minute huddle
- ☐ Review 3–7 key measures (scoreboard)
- ☐ Round: ask the 4 standard questions

- ☐ Capture barriers in an action log
- ☐ Remove/escalate the top barrier of the day
- ☐ Close one loop back to staff ("we heard you—here's the update")
- ☐ Do one coaching touchpoint (2–5 minutes)

Weekly

- ☐ Review repeat barriers + pick one to fix
- ☐ Check staffing patterns (OT, call-outs, breaks, coverage risk)

Monthly

- ☐ Audit 1–2 standards: what's slipping and why

Red Flags (What Not To Do)

Don't confuse LSW with "more tasks." It replaces reactivity with rhythm.

Don't round without follow-up—staff will stop telling you the truth.

Don't track 25 items; pick the critical few and do them consistently.

Don't let "busy" cancel your cadence—busy is when you need it most.

Sidebar: The Three Buckets of Leader Work (and what to protect)

1. **Run Today (Stability):** huddle, staffing, flow, safety risk mitigation

2. **Improve Tomorrow (Removing Friction):** fix one recurring barrier per week

3. **Build People (Capacity):** coaching, recognition, accountability, development

If you only do Bucket 1, you'll stay trapped in the same problems.

Presenting the Concept of Standard Work:

- "This replaces reactivity." We're not adding tasks; we're standardizing the few actions that prevent repeat fires.
- "If it doesn't protect an outcome, it's not on the list." (keeps it lean)
- "20–40 minutes total, spread across the day." (sets a realistic expectation)
- "The payoff is fewer interruptions later." (makes it self-interested in a healthy way)

A Practical Rollout That Usually Lands Well:

Start with only 3 daily items for 2–3 weeks: huddle, rounding (4 questions), action-log follow-up.

Add closed-loop updates once the rhythm is stable.

Keep the weekly barrier review to 15 minutes and focus on the oldest items first.

Chapter 8

Measuring Everything and Managing Nothing

Metrics can be a flashlight or a fog machine. If your dashboard makes people argue about definitions more than outcomes, it's not a dashboard—it's a distraction.

The Friction (What's Happening in Real Life)

Translation: A metric without a decision attached is just a number wearing a nametag.

You have lots of reports—but no one is sure which ones matter.

Leaders ask for "more data" when what they need is a decision.

Staff feel "measured" but not supported; leaders feel accountable but not informed.

Meetings turn into number-reading or spreadsheet-debating instead of solving problems.

Your best people can tell when a metric is being used as a weapon (and they start protecting themselves).

Levity check: if the metric requires a PhD in Excel to explain, it's probably not a frontline-friendly signal.

Why This Matters (Behavior, Reliability, Trust)

People don't change because you show them a number. They change when a number is tied to a clear story: what matters, why it matters, and what we're doing next.

Too many metrics create noise—leaders chase what's loud instead of what's important.

Unclear metrics create cynicism ("They don't know what they're measuring, but they're still mad about it").

Weaponized metrics create hiding and underreporting—exactly the opposite of safety culture.

Right-sized metrics create alignment: teams can see progress and adjust quickly.

The Move (What to Do Instead)

Build a "Small Dashboard" that drives behavior: 3–7 measures max, each with an owner, a target, and a meeting where action happens.

Pick the outcome (what you're ultimately protecting or improving).

Pick 1–2 process measures (the behaviors that drive the outcome).

Pick 1 balancing measure (so you don't fix one thing and break another).

Define each measure in one sentence (so two people can't interpret it two ways).

Assign an owner and an action cadence (who talks about it, where, and how often).

Step-by-Step (The "3–2–1 Dashboard" Method)

Use this when you're drowning in dashboards or launching a new focus area.

3. Outcomes: What three outcomes matter most to this team right now? (Think: safety, experience, workforce, throughput).

2. Drivers Each: For each outcome, what two behaviors/ processes most predict success?

1. Balancer: What could get worse if we push too hard on these? (Example: overtime, delays, staff injuries, patient complaints).

If your team can't connect the metric to something they control, it's a spectator sport. Swap it for a driver measure.

Words You Can Use Monday (Leadership phrases)

Use these as written until they feel like yours. Clear beats clever.

When you need to simplify a dashboard:

"If we could only watch five things that would change behavior this month, what would they be—and why?"

When people debate definitions:

"Let's write the definition in one sentence so we stop arguing and start improving."

When the metric feels punitive:

"This number is a signal, not a grade. We're using it to learn and adjust—not to blame."

When leadership asks for more data:

"Before we pull more reports: what decision will this data help us make?"

When the team needs ownership:

"Who owns this measure, and what's one action we'll try before next week?"

Pocket Checklist

- ☐ Limit to 3–7 measures per team (max).
- ☐ Include 1–2 outcomes, 2–4 drivers, and 1 balancer.
- ☐ Define each measure in one sentence.
- ☐ Display it where people work (not buried in email).
- ☐ Assign an owner for each measure.
- ☐ Set targets that are realistic and time-bound.
- ☐ Review in a meeting that produces actions—not opinions.
- ☐ Tie every "red" to the next step (owner + date).
- ☐ Celebrate "green" with what worked (so it can be repeated).
- ☐ Retire metrics that don't drive behavior.

If You Only Remember One Thing

A metric without ownership is a number. A metric with ownership becomes a behavior change engine.

Chapter 9

Letting Problems Linger Until They Become Personal

In healthcare, problems don't quietly go away. They either get resolved... or they escalate into full-blown conflict. Rapid problem-solving is cultural work.

The Friction (What's Happening in Real Life)

The same issues come up every week (supplies, staffing patterns, handoffs, delays).

People are frustrated—but the only "fix" is a workaround.

Small problems turn into blame ("they never...", "we always...").

You don't have time for a full project, but doing nothing costs more time.

You feel stuck between 'urgent' and 'important' every single day.

Levity check: A workaround is a problem wearing a fake mustache.

Why This Matters (Safety, Experience, Burnout)

Unsolved problems create moral distress—people know the right way but can't do it.

Workarounds increase variation and error risk.

Repeated friction points become "culture" ("That's how it is here").

Rapid problem -solving builds trust: staff sees leadership as responsive and reliable.

The Move (What to Do Instead)

Use a 15–30 minute "Rapid Cycle" approach: define, contain, test, and follow up. Not perfect—better.

Step-by-Step (The 30-Minute Rapid Cycle)

Define the problem in one sentence (no stories, facts + impact).

Contain the risk today (what's the safest temporary step?).

Identify the most likely cause (one, not ten).

Choose one small test of change (PDCA style).

Assign an owner + a check-back time (24–72 hours).

Close the loop and decide: adopt, adapt, or abandon.

The purpose of rapid cycles isn't to be fancy. It's to stop bleeding time and sanity.

Words You Can Use Monday (Leadership phrases)

Use these as written until they feel like yours. Clear beats clever.

To stop the story spiral:

"Let's capture this in one sentence: what happened, where, and what was the impact?"

To contain risk today:

"What's the safest temporary step we can take for the next 24 hours?"

To pick a cause without overanalyzing:

"If we could only test one hypothesis this week, what would it be?"

To choose a small test:

"What's the smallest change we can try by Friday that would tell us if we're on the right track?"

To force follow-through:

"Who owns it, and when are we checking back?"

Pocket Checklist

One-sentence problem statement.
Impact stated (safety/ time/ experience/ staffing).
Containment step for today.
One likely cause (hypothesis).
One small test of change (not a committee).
One owner.
One deadline (24–72 hours).
One place to track it (simple list).
Check back on time.
Close the loop to the team.

If You Only Remember One Thing

Don't wait for a perfect project plan. Run a quick test—then learn your way forward.

Chapter 10

Launching Change Without a Plan to Keep it Alive

Change is easy to announce. Sustaining it is the part where your calendar, staffing, and human nature all conspire against you.

The Friction (What's Happening in Real Life)

You roll out something new... and two weeks later it's back to the old way.

Staff nod in the meeting, then revert under pressure.

Leaders repeatedly remind people, which starts to sound like nagging.

A few exceptions become the rule, and reliability disappears.

Everyone is tired. The appetite for "one more initiative" is gone.

Why This Matters (Reliability and Respect)

Broken change efforts create cynicism ("Here we go again").

Inconsistent practice increases variation and risk.

Leaders get exhausted "policing" instead of leading.

Sustained change protects staff: fewer surprises, less rework, more predictability.

The Move (What to Do Instead)

Sustain change with three anchors: standard, support, and spot-checks. This is how you make the new way the easy way.

Step-By-Step (The 4-Week Sustain Plan)

Week 1: Define the standard in plain language (what 'good' looks like).

Week 1: Remove one barrier (supplies, time, workflow confusion).

Week 2: Train in the workflow (not in a PowerPoint).

Week 2–3: Spot-check with curiosity (not 'gotcha').

Week 3: Share wins and adjustments publicly (make learning visible).

Week 4: Decide what becomes routine (where it lives, who owns it).

Sustainment is not motivation. Sustainment is design.

Words You Can Use Monday (Leadership phrases)

Use these as written until they feel like yours. Clear beats clever.

To set the standard without sounding punitive:

"Here's what 'good' looks like so we're all playing the same game."

To address reversion under pressure:

"When we're busy, we default to old habits. What would make the new way easier in the real workflow?"

To spot-check the right way:

"I'm checking for system issues, not trying to catch people doing something wrong."

To handle exceptions:

"Is this a rare exception—or have we created a loophole that will become the norm?"

To reinforce without nagging:

"Let's review what we learned this week and what we're adjusting."

Pocket Checklist

- ☐ State the standard in one paragraph.
- ☐ Make the standard visible at the point of use.
- ☐ Remove one barrier in week 1.
- ☐ Train in the workflow, not verbally.
- ☐ Create a simple reminder (cue) in the process.
- ☐ Spot-check weekly with curiosity.
- ☐ Share results and lessons weekly.
- ☐ Fix the system before you correct the person.
- ☐ Close loopholes respectfully.
- ☐ Assign a long-term owner.

If You Only Remember One Thing

If the new way requires heroic effort, it won't last. Design the workflow so the right behavior is the default.

Part III

Leading Across the System

Chapter 11

Handoffs - Where Outcomes Die (and How to Fix Them)

When one department is stressed, it's easy to see other departments as obstacles. When they're stressed, they see you the same way. Congratulations—we've built a silo.

And silos rarely announce themselves as silos. They show up as delays, missing information, rework, finger-pointing, and patients who experience the whole thing as waiting, confusion, or "I don't know."

Bad people do not cause most bad days. Bad handoffs cause them.

A handoff is a baton pass. If "done" is not clearly defined, reality fills in the gaps. Usually badly.

When the Problem Wasn't the People

Leadership Moment

One afternoon in the emergency department, I started hearing the same frustration from multiple directions.

The ED nurses were irritated with the imaging department. Imaging was irritated with the ED. Patients were waiting longer than anyone liked, and everyone had a theory about who was to blame.

One nurse said, "Imaging never calls us when they're ready."

Later that day, someone from imaging told me, "The ED sends patients down before they're actually ready."

Both departments were convinced the other one was the problem.

At first glance, it looked like a relationship issue.

But when we slowed down and mapped the actual steps in the process, something became obvious. There was no shared definition of what "ready" meant.

Sometimes the patient had IV access. Sometimes they didn't.
Sometimes consent was complete. Sometimes it wasn't.
Sometimes transport had been arranged. Sometimes it hadn't.

Each department thought the other one was breaking the process.

In reality, there was no clearly defined process to break.

So instead of trying to referee the argument, we brought the teams together and defined a simple term: what "ready for imaging" actually meant.

Once the handoff was clearly defined, the tension between the departments dropped almost immediately.

That experience reinforced something I've seen many times since:

When work moves between departments, problems often surface as conflicts between people.

But the real problem is usually the handoff.

The Friction (What's Happening in Real Life)

Lab, imaging, pharmacy, IT, revenue cycle, and nursing feel like separate worlds with separate priorities.

Information is missing, inconsistent, or lives in too many places.

Nursing says, “They don’t get it.” Other departments say, “They didn’t follow the process.”

The same question gets asked three times by three different people.

Work gets duplicated because no one trusts the upstream work.

Requests bounce, delays multiply, and everyone feels blamed.

The patient experiences the handoff as waiting, confusion, or silence.

Levity check: if your handoff depends on someone “just knowing,” you’ve built a system powered by mind-reading.

Why This Matters (Safety, Flow, Experience, Money)

Most patient delays are handoff problems, not effort problems.

Broken handoffs create rework: calls, clarifications, repeated assessments, and duplicate documentation.

Rework steals capacity, and then we call it a staffing problem.

Cross-department friction drains morale and increases error risk.

Clinical reliability and financial reliability are connected; documentation, timing, and follow-through all affect both.

Clear handoffs reduce conflict because fewer people feel blamed, surprised, or set up to fail.

Leading across departments is not a personality trait. It is a leadership competency.

The Move (What to Do Instead)

Replace "my request to your department" with shared work across a seam.

That means:

- a shared outcome
- a shared definition of done
- shared visibility to the handoff
- and shared ownership of what happens when it breaks

Do not start with

"Who dropped the ball?"

Start with:

"Where is the baton pass failing, and what does done need to mean on both sides?"

Step-by-Step (The Handoff Alignment Huddle)

Use this to fix one high-pain handoff in 20–30 minutes.

Step 1: Start with the shared outcome

Name the outcome both sides care about:

- patient flow
- safety
- readiness
- timeliness
- patient experience
- reduced rework

If the only goal is "get my department what I need," the meeting will drift into turf protection.

Step 2: Name constraints on both sides

Ask:

"What is hard on your side that we may not see?"

What timing, staffing, regulatory, technology, or workflow realities are shaping this?

This is not an excuse collection. This is system understanding.

Step 3: Map the handoff in 5–7 steps

Keep it simple. Just enough to see where the baton pass fails.

Examples:

- clinic to test
- ED to inpatient
- OR to PACU
- imaging to the unit
- discharge to follow-up

Step 4: Pick one failure point

Do not fix the whole enterprise in one meeting.

Choose the seam that causes the most confusion, delay, or rework.

Step 5: Write the definition of done

Before the baton can pass, what must be true every time?

Examples:

- Orders signed and visible in the agreed location
- patient prep complete
- timing confirmed
- escalation contact identified

- special needs flagged
- required documentation complete

If "done" is fuzzy, blame will fill the space.

Step 6: Define the standard

Agree on:

- Who owns the baton at each step
- where the information lives
- When it must happen
- How the receiver confirms it is complete
- This is where reliability begins.

Step 7: Add closed-loop confirmation

The receiving team confirms:

- They got it
- It is complete
- Or something is missing
- No silent assumptions. No, hoping it made it through the day.

Step 8: Build the contingency

Ask:

- What do we do today if something is missing, incomplete, or urgent?
- This prevents panic and finger-pointing.

Step 9: Pilot for two weeks

Run the new handoff standard for two weeks. Review what improved, what failed, and what still creates rework.
Revise once, then standardize.

Start small. One handoff fixed creates more flow than ten meetings about communication.

Departments rarely fail each other because people don't care.
They fail each other when the seam between them is undefined.

The Leadership Phrases

Use these as written until they feel like yours. Clear beats clever.

To shift from blame to shared work:

"We're on the same side. Let's define the shared outcome and the handoff that's breaking."

"This isn't a people problem first; it's a handoff problem. Let's define 'done' on both sides."

To surface constraints respectfully:

"What's hard on your side that we may not see?"

"What constraints are shaping this step today?"

To define ownership clearly:

"At this step, who owns the baton, and what does 'done' mean?"

"Before we hand this off, what must be true every time?"

To reduce rework:

"Where is the single source of truth for this information?"

"Let's agree on one standard request format, so we stop reworking this."

To require closed-loop communication:

"I need a confirmation so we know this didn't get lost in the day."

"How will the receiver confirm this is complete?"

To manage missing information without drama:

"We're missing _____. Here's the contingency for today, and here's how we prevent it tomorrow."

To reinforce system thinking:

"When the handoff is clean, the day is calmer. This is how we protect patients and staff."

"Fix the pathway, not just the frustration."

Red Flags (What Not to Do)

- Don't treat another department as a vendor rather than a partner in shared work.
- Don't let "communication issues" stay vague; map the actual handoff.
- Don't fix everything at once.
- Don't rely on memory, hallway conversations, or heroics.
- Don't keep correcting people when the process is still unclear.
- Don't assume shared responsibility means no one owns the baton.

Pocket Checklist

- Choose one handoff (high-pain, high-volume).
- Write the definition of done (5–8 items max).
- Define where info lives (one source of truth).
- Set the timing trigger (when it must occur).
- Require closed-loop confirmation.
- Create a missing-info contingency.
- Assign a joint owner (one on each side).
- Pilot for 2 weeks.
- Fix the process before correcting people.
- Standardize once it works.

Chapter 12

Flow Over Silos—Managing Bottlenecks Like a Pro

If you hear "We're full" in one area while another is oddly quiet, that's usually not capacity. That's flow. Flow is leadership work.

The Friction (What's Happening in Real Life)

Days swing between chaos and idle time with no predictability.

One step backs up the whole pathway (beds, imaging slots, transport, pharmacy turnaround, discharge barriers).

Departments optimize locally ("We met our numbers") while the patient journey stalls.

Staff feel like they're sprinting, but outcomes don't improve.

The same bottleneck keeps popping up—and everyone points somewhere else.

Levity check: if your system were a freeway, we'd all be standing around arguing whose lane is moving the slowest.

Why This Matters (Throughput, Workforce, Patient Experience)

Flow problems create waiting, and waiting creates risk (clinical + emotional).

When flow is broken, staff do more work with less impact (classic burnout fuel).

The bottleneck controls output. Improving non-bottlenecks often changes nothing.

Flow-based leadership reduces conflict because it focuses on the pathway rather than the department.

The Move (What to Do Instead)

Manage the constraint (the bottleneck) and protect the pathway. Use a simple flow playbook: identify, exploit, buffer, and trigger.

Step-By-Step (The 4-Step Constraint Playbook)

Find the constraint: where do patients or workers wait the longest (today, not in theory)?

Protect it: ensure the constraint is never waiting on inputs (orders, transport, supplies, staffing).

Create a small buffer: a ready queue that prevents starvation (but not a giant pile of work).

Set triggers: when the constraint is at risk, you activate pre-planned actions (not panic).

Common Hospital Constraints (Look Here First)

Discharge process (transport, meds-to-bed, follow-up appointments, SNF placement)

Diagnostics (imaging slots, lab turnaround, EKG availability)

Procedure start times (OR/ Endo readiness, consents, pre-op completion)

Bed assignment/ cleaning (EVS timing, admissions batching)

Pharmacy verification/ dispense (especially on weekends/ evenings)

Words You Can Use Monday (Leadership phrases)

Use these as written until they feel like yours. Clear beats clever.

To reframe the problem as flow:

"Let's stop debating departments. Where does the patient journey get stuck—step by step?"

To identify the constraint quickly:

"Where are we waiting the most right now, and what's causing that wait?"

To protect the bottleneck:

"What does the constraint need so it never waits on us?"

To set triggers without drama:

"If we hit _____, we activate _____."

To avoid local optimization:

"Even if we're 'green' here, is the patient moving? If not, we fix the pathway."

Pocket Checklist

- Define the pathway (start → finish).
- Name the constraint (where work waits).
- Protect the constraint (inputs ready).
- Create a small buffer (ready queue).
- Set a trigger threshold (when to act).
- Pre-plan 2–3 actions when triggered.
- Track one pathway measure (not department-only).
- Meet briefly at the seam (10–15 minutes).
- Fix the constraint first; then recheck the pathway.
- Repeat weekly until stable.

Chapter 13

Governance That Executes—Committees That Decide

A committee that only discusses is a pressure-release valve, not a decision engine. If meetings don't produce decisions, the work leaks into hallways, texts, and late-night emails.

The Friction (What's Happening in Real Life)

Translation: If the committee can't decide, it's a discussion group. That's fine—just don't call it governance.

Meetings are packed, but action is vague ("We should...", "Let's look into...").

Decisions drift to after the meeting—or never happen at all.

Same topics return monthly with no progress.

People leave confused about who owns what.

Escalations are inconsistent, so problems either fester or explode.

Levity check: if your committee's main deliverable is "awareness," you've created an expensive newsletter.

Why This Matters (Speed, Accountability, Trust)

Governance is how strategy becomes work. Weak governance produces random work.

When decisions drift, staff experience leadership as indecisive or disconnected.

Clear authority prevents turf wars and prevents 'shadow decisions.'

Execution-ready governance reduces meeting load because fewer things need re-discussing.

The Move (What to Do Instead)

Turn committees into execution engines using four non-negotiables: charter, decisions, action log, and escalation path.

Step-by-Step (The Committee Reset in One Meeting)

State the purpose in one sentence (why this committee exists).

Clarify authority: what it can decide, recommend, or escalate.

Define 3–5 measures that the committee is accountable for moving.

Use an agenda that forces decisions (not updates).

Maintain a live action log: decision, owner, due date, status.

End every meeting by reading commitments out loud.

Define escalation triggers (when items must move up).

The Agenda That Prevents Drift (Use This)

1) Safety/quality signals (5 min) — only what changed

2) Scoreboard review (10 min) — red/yellow only

3) Decisions needed today (20 min) — make the call

4) Action log review (10 min) — oldest items first

5) Escalations (5 min) — decide pathways

6) Close: read commitments + due dates (2 min)

Words You Can Use Monday (Leadership phrases)

Use these as written until they feel like yours. Clear beats clever.

To force a decision:

"Is this a decision, a recommendation, or information? If it's a decision point, what are the options?"

To stop endless discussion:

"We've discussed. Now we choose. What decision are we making today?"

To require ownership:

"Who owns the next step, and what's the due date?"

To prevent 'parking lot purgatory':

"If it's important, it gets an owner and a date. If not, we drop it."

To handle disagreement cleanly:

"We can disagree and still decide. What's the best decision for outcomes right now?"

To escalate appropriately:

"This is outside our authority. Here's the escalation with the recommendation and rationale."

Pocket Checklist

- Charter: purpose + authority + membership.
- Define what you decide, recommend, and inform.
- 3–5 measures the committee owns.
- Agenda includes a 'decisions' section.
- Live action log (decision/ owner/ due date).
- Oldest actions reviewed first.
- Commitments read out loud at the end.
- Escalation triggers defined.
- Minutes should capture decisions and actions, not transcripts.
- If no decisions/ actions are made, cancel the meeting.

Mini Tool: One-Page Committee Action Log

Topic | Decision/Action | Owner | Due Date | Status (G/Y/R) | Escalation Needed (Y/N) | Notes

If You Only Remember One Thing

Committees exist to produce decisions and follow-through. If that's not happening, redesign the meeting—not the people.

Chapter 14

Communication That Cuts Through Noise

In healthcare, silence is not neutral. Silence gets filled with rumors, fear, and creative writing. Communicate early, clearly, and consistently—especially when you don't have all the answers yet.

The Friction (What's Happening in Real Life)

Translation: If you have to say it five times, that's not over-communicating. That's leadership.

People hear five different versions of the same message, depending on whom they talk to.

Frontline staff feel surprised by changes that leadership feels were 'communicated.'

Rumors spread faster than the actual plan.

Leaders over-explain (to reduce anxiety) and accidentally create more confusion.

Email becomes a substitute for clarity—and nobody reads it anyway.

Levity check: if your message needs three follow-up emails to explain, it wasn't a message. It was a novel.

Why This Matters (Trust, Compliance, Calm)

Inconsistent messaging creates distrust and resistance—even if the change is reasonable.

Clear messaging reduces anxiety; anxiety is what fuels rumor cycles.

Communication is how you create line-of-sight: what's changing, why, and what to do today.

Consistent communication protects leaders, too—fewer side conversations, fewer misunderstandings.

The Move (What to Do Instead)

Use a repeatable 4-part message every time: **Why → What → What stays the same → What you need to do now**.

Step-by-Step (The 4-Part Message)

Why: the purpose (patient safety, experience, workforce, reliability).

What: the change in plain language (one paragraph).

What stays the same: anchor the team (reduce threat response).

Now: what you need people to do today/this week (specific actions).

If you don't know something yet, say so—and give a time when you will know. Uncertainty with the timeline beats silence every time.

Message Channels That Work (Use 2, Not 6)

One spoken channel: huddle/rounding/leader cascade (same words)

One written channel: short email/poster with the same 4 parts

Optional: FAQ for complex changes (one page max)

Words You Can Use Monday (Leadership phrases)

Use these as written until they feel like yours. Clear beats clever.

When you don't have all the answers:

"Here's what we know today, here's what we don't know yet, and here's when you'll get the next update."

To stop rumor cycles:

"I'm hearing multiple versions. Here's the single accurate message, and here's where updates will live."

To translate strategy into action:

"This matters because _____. Starting today, here's what changes in our workflow: _____."

To reduce fear:

"What stays the same is _____. What's changing is _____. The goal is _____."

To hold consistency across leaders:

"Use this exact language so staff gets one message, not five interpretations."

To close with clarity:

"If you remember one thing: _____. If you do one thing today: _____."

Pocket Checklist

Use the 4-part message (Why/What/Same/Now).

Keep the 'What' to one paragraph.

Name what you don't know yet + when you'll update.

Use one spoken channel + one written channel.

Give a single source of truth for updates.

Repeat the message (consistency beats novelty).

Align leader cascade wording (no freelancing).

Address the rumor directly and calmly.

Ask: "What did you hear?" to test understanding.

End with one action people must take.

Mini Tool: One-Page Message Template

WHY (purpose):

WHAT (change):

WHAT STAYS THE SAME (anchors):

WHAT TO DO NOW (actions):

NEXT UPDATE (date/time + where):

If You Only Remember One Thing

Your communication isn't what you said. It's what people heard. Use a repeatable structure until the message sticks.

Part IV

Leadership Maturity

Chapter 15

Tight-End vs Loose-End Leadership

The rope you're holding

Leadership is a lot like holding a rope.

Some days you need the tight end—closer to the work, more structure, faster correction—because reliability matters and variation is expensive.

Other days, you need the loose end—more space, more ownership, more learning—because growth requires autonomy.

The mistake isn't choosing one end. The mistake is using the same end for every situation, then calling it "my style."

The principle that keeps you honest

Tight on the WHAT and WHY. Flexible on the HOW.

Even when you lead on the loose end, you're not hands-off—you're standards-on.

What the two ends look like

Tight end leadership (High structure)

On the tight end, you reduce variation and create reliability:

Standards, checklists, deadlines

Short feedback loops (daily/ weekly)

Rapid correction when performance drifts

Decisions are centralized when needed

Best used when:

Risk is high (patient safety, regulatory exposure)

There is a clearly "right way."

The team/process is new or inconsistent

Conditions are urgent or unstable

Watch out: Tight leadership without trust feels like control.

Loose end leadership (High autonomy)

On the loose end, you create ownership and build capacity:

- Outcome + guardrails, flexible methods
- Coaching questions > instructions
- Decisions pushed closest to the work
- Learning loops (experiment, review, refine)

Best used when:

- Risk is low to moderate
- The team is competent and aligned
- You need innovation or problem-solving
- You're developing leaders and succession

Watch out: Loose leadership without clarity feels like neglect.

The 3-question grip check

Use this quick tool to choose the right end before you react.

Risk: If this goes wrong, what is the cost?

Maturity: How proven is the process/team?

Clarity: *Do we know the right way—or are we discovering it?*

Rule of thumb

High risk + low maturity + high clarity → Tight end

Low risk + high maturity + lower clarity → Loose end

Self-assessment: What end do you default to?

How to take it

Rate each statement 1–5

1 = rarely true • 3 = sometimes • 5 = almost always true

Tight-end tendencies

When things feel messy, my first move is to add structure (rules, steps, deadlines).

I prefer to standardize first before delegating broadly.

I feel responsible for catching problems early, even if it means staying close to the details.

I'm quick to correct variation ("this is not the way we do it").

I'm most comfortable when expectations are explicit and measurable.

Under pressure, I tighten oversight (more check-ins, more direction).

Tight Score = total (1–6)

Loose-end tendencies

I define the outcome and let the team design how.

I'm comfortable with different approaches as long as the results are met.

I use questions more than instructions to develop people.

I push decisions as close to the work as possible whenever possible.

I treat mistakes as data for learning, not just noncompliance.

Under pressure, I try to protect autonomy and avoid overcorrecting.

Loose Score = total (7–12)

Interpret your pattern

Tight high / Loose low: You build reliability. Watch for overdependence on you.

Loose high / Tight low: You build capacity. Watch for drift and variation.

Both high: You can shift ends. Watch for inconsistency if you don't explain the shift.

Both low: You may be avoiding discomfort or unclear on authority—start by tightening the WHAT/WHY.

Your stress (circle one)

I grip tighter under pressure (control, directives, frequent follow-ups).

I let go under pressure (less follow-through, unclear expectations).

That's your default. Awareness is step one. Choice is step two.

Leader language that prevents whiplash

When you shift ends, say it out loud. It lowers anxiety and preserves trust.

When tightening:

"Because the risk is high and the standard is clear, we're leading this on the tight end for the next 30 days."

"This is not optional because the cost of variation is too high."

When loosening:

"You've proven reliability. The standard stays tight—now you own improvements to the process."

"I'm stepping back on the how. I'll stay close to outcomes and barriers."

Examples you can steal

Example 1: Medication reconciliation (Tight → slight loosen)

Situation: Admission medication reconciliation is inconsistent. Risk is high. The right way is known. Grip: Start with the tight end.

What tight looks like (first 30 days):

Non-negotiable expectation (by time of day/within X hours)

Checklist embedded in workflow (and roles clarified)

Frequent auditing + quick feedback

Clear escalation path for barriers

Leader language:

"Because the risk is high and the standard is clear, we're on the tight end for 30 days. Reliability first."

When you loosen: Once it's stable, the staff can describe the process without guessing.

What loosen looks like: Spot checks instead of constant audits; the team owns workflow improvements.

Example 2: OR block release compliance (Tight on the policy, loose on solutions)

Situation: Block time isn't being released, access suffers, and utilization underperforms. Policy exists. Compliance is inconsistent.
Grip: Tight end on the rules, loose end on improvement ideas.

Tight on the WHAT (non-negotiables):

Policy enforced as written (e.g., 7-day release rule)

Transparent reporting (utilization + release compliance)

Defined accountability steps

Loose on the HOW (team solves it):

Surgeons/OR leaders propose practical triggers (vacation rule, confirm-or-release automation, etc.)

Leader language:

"We're tight on access and fairness. How we get there is flexible—but the outcome isn't."

Example 3: Launching a Clinical Flex Team (Loose → Tight → Loose)

Situation: You're designing a staffing model to cover absences without destabilizing units. Early work needs buy-in; later work needs reliability.

Grip: Loose → Tight → Loose

Phase 1 (Loose): Design and ownership

Outcome + guardrails (scope, training minimums, scheduling rules, pay rules)

Front-line input shapes workflow

Phase 2 (Tight): Standardize and stabilize

Training/competency checklist

Clear activation criteria

Weekly operational review for 8–12 weeks

Phase 3 (Loose): Optimize and grow leaders

Team proposes improvements

Review cadence relaxes as reliability holds

Leader language:

"We're in learning mode first. Then we tighten the rope to stabilize. Once it's solid, we loosen again so leaders grow."

Example 4: Data request intake (Tight on intake, loose on insights)

Situation: Requests arrive at random; definitions vary; trust in the data is low.

Grip:

Tight on intake and definitions; loose on analysis format.

Tight:

One front door intake process

Required fields (purpose, decision, owner, definition, due date)

Prioritization rules

Loose:

Analysts and teams prototype visuals and iterate

Focus on decision usefulness, not perfection

Leader language:

"We're tight on clarity and transparency. We're loose on format. The goal is better decisions."

Closing: *The goal isn't control or freedom—it's maturity*

You're not trying to become a "tight leader" or a "loose leader." You're trying to become a leader who can choose the right end, move along the rope without drama, and explain the shift in a way that preserves trust.

- Tight end builds reliability
- Loose ends build capacity
- Great leaders build both—on purpose.

Chapter 16

Run Your Unit Like a COO: The SPOCK Leadership Model

Run your unit like an operator, not just a responder.

One of the most useful lessons I took from Baldrige was this: results are outputs of a system. They result from the combined effects of strategy, people, operations, competence, and the use and transfer of knowledge.

That matters for nurse leaders. If we only manage the schedule and solve today's disruptions, we stay reactive. If we run the unit like an operation within the organization, we start building reliability that withstands turnover, pressure, and personalities.

SPOCK is the mental model I use to keep that work organized: Strategy, People, Operations, Competence, and Knowledge Management & Transfer.

- *Strategy*
- *People*
- *Operations*
- *Competence*
- *Knowledge Management & Transfer*

The Unit COO Mindset

A strong nurse leader should be able to answer five questions at any given time:

Where are we going?

Do we have the right people, in the right roles, with the right support?

How does the work run, and where does it break?

What capabilities are we building next?

What are we learning, and how are we making that learning stick beyond one person?

1) Strategy

Strategy is "How we win" for patients, staff, and the organization

What it means for a nursing leader:

Strategy is not the organization's strategic plan on a poster. Strategy is your unit's direction translated into priorities, targets, and decisions, yet aligned with the organization's strategic plan.

Strategy deliverables (what a strong unit always has)

A. The Unit "True North" (1 sentence)

- Why we exist (patient/community impact) – the mission
- How we'll be known (quality, experience, reliability) – for example, top percentile performance, five-star CMS rating
- What we refuse to compromise (safety, dignity, standards)

B. A short list of annual strategic aims (3–5) Examples:

- Reduce harm (falls, pressure injuries, medication administration defects)
- Improve flow (Length of stay, throughput, discharge by noon)
- Stabilize staffing (retention, sick time, vacancy)
- Strengthen patient experience
- Develop next-level leaders

C. The "stop doing" list

- If everything is a priority, nothing is. Your stop list protects focus and reduces staff fatigue.
- COO-level strategy questions (ask monthly)
- What are the 3 outcomes we must deliver this quarter?
- What are the constraints (FTE, beds, supplies, training) and how are we designing around them?
- What would we stop doing if we had to cut effort by 10% without lowering safety?
- What is the biggest strategic risk to performance, and what's our mitigation?

2) People

People systems create culture; culture creates results

Baldrige explicitly focuses on workforce capability and engagement as a driver of performance (not a "nice to have").

What it means for a nursing leader:

Your job is to build the conditions where great people can do great work—consistently.

People fundamentals (what to build)

A. Role Clarity

- "What I own" vs "what I influence."
- Visible decision rights: what staff can decide, what charge can decide, what manager decides, etc.

B. Staffing Integrity

- A staffing plan that matches demand patterns (not averages)
- A plan for variability (surges, call-outs, long leaves)

- A fairness standard (transparent assignment + escalation)

C. **Engagement by design (not by luck)**
- Recognition tied to values and behaviors
- Listening system: rounding, huddles, pulse surveys, skip-levels
- Psychological safety: staff can surface defects without punishment

3. Operations

Operations are the "how" that turns effort into reliability

Baldrige operations thinking focuses on managing work as processes, so results don't rely on individual heroics.

What it means for a nursing leader: If you can't describe your unit's key processes, you can't improve them—and you can't hold them.

The 7 "must-control" nursing processes

Pick the ones that fit your unit, but most units have some version of:

Patient intake/admission flow

Handoffs and communication

Medication management (including reconciliation)

Discharge planning and coordination

Escalation/rapid response/decompensation pathway (avoid failure to rescue)

Staffing and assignment workflow

Daily management system (huddle → actions → follow-up)

Operational discipline: standard work + flexibility

Standardize what must be reliable (safety, compliance, handoffs)

Flex what must be adaptive (patient needs, individualized care, individualized staff needs)

4. Competence

Competence is your unit's ability to perform today—and improve tomorrow.

This is where many units fall short: they rely on experience to carry capability. Strong leaders develop competence on purpose.

What competence means here:

Clinical competence (safe, evidence-based care, accurate policies)

Operational competence (flow, prioritization, escalation)

Improvement in competence (problem-solving, data use)

Leadership competence (coaching, accountability, communication, continuous improvement)

5. Knowledge Management & Transfer

If knowledge only lives in people's heads, your unit is fragile.

When your best charge nurse retires, does excellence retire with her?

Baldrige explicitly elevates "Measurement, Analysis, and Knowledge Management" as a core performance category—because learning must be captured and transferred to sustain results.

High-performing units do not just work well; they excel. They remember well.

What it means for a nursing leader:

Your unit shouldn't "relearn" the same lessons every year. You need a system to capture, share, and safeguard institutional knowledge—especially during turnover. If you fix a throughput issue this spring and struggle with it again next fall, you don't have a performance problem — you have a knowledge transfer problem.

Knowledge you must manage (4 types)

- Clinical knowledge (guidelines, pathways, safety practices)
- Operational knowledge (how the unit runs, escalation rules, flow)
- Improvement knowledge (what we tried, what worked, what didn't)
- Relationship knowledge (who to call, how to coordinate across departments)

Leader Check

- If someone stepped into your role tomorrow, would they inherit clarity — or chaos?
- If your answer is chaos, that's not a character flaw. It's a system gap.
- And system gaps are solvable.

The Unit COO Scorecard

If you want one page to run your unit like a business, use this structure:

Strategy: 3–5 Priorities + Targets + Stop List

People: *staffing stability + engagement + development pipeline*

Operations: *top 5 processes + reliability measures + flow*

Competence: *competency map + charge/preceptor dept*

Knowledge: *playbook + onboarding + AARs + two-deep coverage*

Baldrige as a Nursing Superpower

The Baldrige journey reveals something many leaders feel but can't articulate: results are intentionally designed. When nursing leaders develop strong systems around these five fundamentals, they move beyond just "surviving the week" and begin delivering excellence deliberately. The SPOCK model—because when nursing operations get loud, you need Spock-level logic: calm, clear priorities, and decisions that follow the data.

This book exists to give nursing leaders real-life, proven tools for challenging work: imperfect systems, real people, and real constraints. It's not a makeover; it's a plan. You will make mistakes—because you're human. The goal is fewer preventable errors and faster recovery when they happen. This isn't about changing your personality; it's about building a practice. And the good news? Imperfect systems can be improved—one clear step at a time.

If you only keep five things:

Find the real problem (the loud one is often just the symptom).

Run your unit like a COO: use the SPOCK model to organize the work.

Make ownership visible: *who owns what by when.*

Standardize what must be repeatable and reliable; coach what must grow.

Close loops out loud. Trust is built in follow-through.

Closure: *Leading in the Fog: Decision Principles*

When the future is uncertain, we rely on our core values as our guide: Trust, Teamwork, and Transparency. We can't always wait for certainty to take action. We won't always have all the data.

So we move forward anyway—one clear step at a time. Don't mistake discomfort for danger. Keep making progress. Use decision principles to guide the next steps.

Decision Principles for Leading in the Fog

1. **Anchor to values first.**

   When the "right answer" isn't obvious, choose the option most aligned with Trust, Teamwork, and Transparency.

2. **Protect safety and dignity—always.**

   Patient safety and a psychologically safe workplace are non-negotiable. If an option increases risk, pause and redesign.

3. **Take the next best step, not the perfect step.**

   Progress beats paralysis. Make a decision that moves us forward and can be adjusted as we learn.

4. **Decide faster when it's reversible; slow down when it's not.**

   If we can undo it, decide, learn, and iterate. If it's hard to reverse, slow down, involve others, and pressure-test assumptions.

5. **Get "enough" information—then act.**

   Gather the minimum data needed to reduce major risk, clarify tradeoffs, and choose a direction. Don't wait for total certainty.

6. **Name assumptions out loud.**

   Say what we believe is true, what we don't know yet, and what would change our mind. Unspoken assumptions still drive decisions.

7. **Make tradeoffs explicit.**

   Every decision costs something—time, money, capacity, goodwill. Be clear about what we're optimizing for and what we're willing to accept.

8. **Involve the right people early.**

   If a decision impacts others, bring them in—especially those closest to the patient and those doing the work. Better context creates better decisions.

9. **Bias toward mission and patient impact.**

   When options compete, choose the path that most improves access, quality, and experience for our rural community.

10. **Communicate the why, the what, and the when.**

    Transparency lowers anxiety. Share the rationale, what happens next, and how feedback will be handled—even if the answer is, "We're still learning."

11. **Build feedback loops and checkpoints.**

    Decide, act, measure, and adjust. Set a review point—24 hours, one week, or 30 days—so we don't drift.

12. **Own it—and learn fast.**

    Accountability means we stand behind decisions, correct quickly when reality proves us wrong, and share what we learn so the organization gets smarter.

Leading in the fog isn't about being certain. It's about being clear, values-anchored, and willing to learn in motion.

Leading When the Work is Hard

If you've made it this far, you already know something important about healthcare leadership:

The work is messy.

There will always be more problems than time,

more expectations than resources,

and more decisions than certainty.

Some days you will walk into a room and feel the emotional weather immediately: tension, fatigue, frustration, urgency. On those days, leadership can feel like carrying the weight of everything.

But that is not the job.

The job is to create clarity when the system is under stress.

It is to slow the moment down long enough for people to think again.

It is to help teams move from reaction to problem-solving.

It is to make ownership visible, so work actually moves forward.

And over time, it is to design systems where the right actions become the easiest actions.

You will still make mistakes. Every leader does.

The goal is not perfection.

The goal is fewer preventable messes, faster recovery when they happen, and a team that grows steadier because you lead more steadily.

If you take only a few ideas with you, take these:

- Find the real problem.
- Make ownership visible.
- Fix the pathway, not just the frustration.

- Close loops out loud.

When the room speeds up, slow it down until the work becomes clear again.

Healthcare leadership will always be demanding. It is also meaningful because every improvement in the system makes it easier for patients and caregivers to thrive.

  - So keep learning.
  - Keep adjusting.
  - Keep building better systems.

And when the work feels overwhelming, remember this:

You do not have to have all the answers.

You do have to help the team think clearly enough to take the next right step.

Carry This with You

Healthcare leadership is demanding. When the day gets loud and the system gets messy, return to the few practices that keep work moving forward:

- ***Regulate yourself first.***

  When the room speeds up, slow yourself down. Teams take emotional cues from their leaders.

- ***Create clarity.***

  Define the problem in one sentence. Ask: What is true? What matters? What is the next step?

- ***Make ownership visible.***

  Every action needs an owner and a due time. If ownership is unclear, progress stalls.

- ***Separate context from accountability.***

  Barriers are real, but they do not replace ownership.

- ***Fix the pathway, not just the frustration.***

  Most recurring problems are system problems. Map the process before blaming people.

- ***Run the day with rhythm.***

  Huddles, leader standard work, and rapid problem-solving keep the system steady.

- ***Protect the seams between teams.***

  Most delays and conflicts happen at handoffs. Define what "done" means before passing the baton.

- ***Decide at the right level.***

  Push decisions as close to the work as possible, but stay tight on standards and outcomes.

- ***Communicate early and often.***

  Silence creates rumors. Clear structure lowers anxiety.

- ***Close loops out loud.***

  Trust grows when people see that concerns raised are acted on.

When the Work Feels Overwhelming

Remember This:

Leadership is not about having all the answers.

Leadership is about helping people think clearly enough to take the next right step.

www.ingramcontent.com/pod-product-compliance
Lightning Source LLC
LaVergne TN
LVHW100148061126
851857LV00010B/303

* 9 7 9 8 2 5 6 1 2 3 7 9 6 *